ALS

A Respiratory Perspective

KIPLING A. JACKSON

2018

ISBN: 9781549853166

Printed in the United States of America
FIRST EDITION, 2018

WWW.KIPLINGAJACKSON.COM

Table of Contents

Foreword 7
Chapter 1: ALS and Me 11
Chapter 2: Eating and Swallowing Problems in ALS 23
Chapter 3: Respiratory Failure in ALS 29
Chapter 4: To Trach or not to Trach 39
Chapter 5: After the Tracheostomy 47
Chapter 6: Passive Respiratory Therapy 57
Chapter 7: Active Respiratory Therapy 63
Chapter 8: Road Trips and Redundancy 69
Chapter 9: Close Encounters of the Kip Kind 75
Afterword 85
Works Cited 89

Robin, I couldn't have done this without you. I love you!

Foreword

Before we begin, let's get the disclaimers out of the way. First, I'm not a medical doctor, nor do I play one on TV. Second, this book is not a substitute for medical advice and should not be taken as such. Next, if you suspect you have ALS or have any questions about the disease, please consult your physician or neurologist. If you're interested in the tracheostomy or have any questions about trach maintenance, talk with your respiratory therapist, pulmonologist, or ENT doctor. Finally, if you're experiencing an emergency, drop the frappin' book and call 911!

In 2015, one of my respiratory therapists asked me to do a presentation on ALS for that year's state respiratory symposium. ALS is such a rare disease that little education circulates among medical professionals. Well, I said "yes" immediately – I'm ready to oblige when offered any pertinent opportunity to speak on my disease. At the time, I had been trached and vented for a year and living with the disease for three years. After the presentation, one of my other respiratory therapists told me she had received a lot of positive feedback on my presentation and suggested I write a book using the material from my appearance. So, here I am two years later with the finished product.

Fear seems to permeate the air every time mechanical ventilation or the tracheostomy is mentioned. Contributing to this fear is the lack of information available to help the ALS patient make an informed decision about extending their life with these techniques. Since I have now been living with mechanical ventilation and the trach for three years and five months, I want to share with my fellow ALS patients and their families the story of the personal respiratory struggles I've been through.

I've been deliberately vague about some issues. This book is designed to nudge you in the right direction, to help you open a dialogue with the appropriate medical professionals, not as a how-to manual in a time of crisis.

ALS is one of those diseases in which every person will trail-blaze their own path through the duration of it. For some patients, ALS starts with weakness in the legs; for others, the disease starts with unexplained cramps in a hand. I know of a few mechanically ventilated and trached patients who still eat and drink, and others who can still communicate verbally. Each distinct pathway creates a different story – I can only tell you mine.

Kipling A. Jackson

9/10/17

Chapter 1 | ALS and Me

I have lived with ALS or "Lou Gehrig's Disease" for five years now. ALS stands for *amyotrophic lateral sclerosis*. According to the ALS Association, ALS

> is a progressive neurodegenerative disease that affects nerve cells in the brain and the spinal cord... Motor neurons reach from the brain to the spinal cord and from the spinal cord to the muscles throughout the body. The progressive degeneration of the motor neurons in ALS eventually leads to their demise. When the motor neurons die, the ability of the brain to initiate and control

> muscle movement is lost. With voluntary muscle action progressively affected, people may lose the ability to speak, eat, and breathe...[1]

If a ventilator isn't used, the patient will die of respiratory failure. ALS is a terminal disease.

Every patient has experienced fasciculations (uncontrolled muscle twitching). This symptom alone is, in some cases, benign, but when the phenomenon is followed by muscle weakness, it raises a red flag leading toward a diagnosis of ALS.

In fact, the first symptom that presented itself to me was severe twitching in my left index finger. I thought I was cool; I thought I was special. It was the perfect conversation piece at parties.

"Well, I'm glad you're doing well in the stock market, and your 401k is at an all-time high. You must be very proud." I'm bored with the gentleman at this point. Spotting my wife across the room, rolling my eyes, I then ask the man with all the enthusiasm I can muster, "Hey, looky here, can your finger do this? No, don't pull it just watch." Oohs and ahs emanate from the crowd. Everybody looks at each other amazed. Then they finally break into a glorious round of applause. I'm so overcome by emotion that I have no choice but to take a bow.

Little did I know what this simple tremor in my finger would lead to. I did have a premonition that something might be wrong. When I suffered a concussion after experiencing several falls, I knew a serious problem existed. Thus, began a long, tedious road to a diagnosis – eight months would pass before I received the verdict.

No diagnostic test exists for sporadic ALS, the type of ALS I have. Consequently, the journey becomes a lengthy process of elimination – are there any tumors, lesions, or abnormalities in your brain? No. Are there any irregularities in your spinal fluid? No. Could you have any heavy metal present, which could result in neurotoxins attacking your brain? No. Do you have Lyme Disease? No. Is there any delay in the speed of the signals your motor neurons are sending to the muscles and nerves? Yes. Are you experiencing fasciculations and weakness in your muscles? Yes.

My first neurologist comes into the room and said, "Mr. Jackson, there's a strong possibility that you have ALS. There is no cure." Then silence. I searched the good doctor's face for any sign of compassion. Nothing. "Life expectancy with the disease is two to five years." *Now,* did I get any sympathy? The neurologist's expression didn't give: it was as cold as the grave I'd be buried in.

I thought, Seriously, is that it? Have you nothing more to say?

The doc could have at least offered me a stick of Juicy Fruit® or even a breath mint – a Tic Tac®, perhaps? Alas, it was not to be. Instead, I got stuck with a bunch of pamphlets about ALS – stuff I knew by heart from my extensive internet research.

Oh, for me? A bunch of useless pamphlet? You shouldn't have. Uh – thanks anyway.

Look, doc, shake my hand, look me in the eye, and tell me, "Good luck with that, Mr. Jackson," instead of wasting all your money on those dreadful handouts. Save a tree or two; it will have more of a positive impact on humankind than how you treated me.

We need to bridge this gap of bad doctor-patient relationships. I think doctors should start offering the patient a voucher for one free chocolate pudding from the hospital cafeteria upon receiving a diagnosis of a terminal disease. Whipped cream would cost you extra, though.

What did the neurologist mean that there was a "strong possibility" that I had ALS? Remember, a test for sporadic ALS hasn't been established yet. But that tentative diagnosis was hard for me to accept. I'm an analytical guy who lives in a world where two answers exist: the right one and the wrong one. There is no gray area.

The first neurologist presented the news to me without collecting all the information, which was a big problem for me. I want to examine *all* the evidence to back up any assertion, especially if it concerns me. Since there are several ailments that mimic the symptoms of ALS, I thought the doctor should have left no stone unturned before concluding that I had a terminal condition. A lumbar puncture to analyze my spinal fluids wasn't performed. I was not pleased.

Immediately after leaving the office, I scheduled an appointment to get a second opinion. The second neurologist did a thorough medical work-up including the lumbar puncture. The results were negative; no abnormalities were present in my spinal fluid. For the second time, I was told the data pointed to ALS.

No worries, first neurologist, the joke was on me. I was the one who chose to endure the second battery of tests, only to be told the same thing. Every single day proves your educated guess was correct, since I'm now totally paralyzed, tube-fed, trached, and ventilator dependent. But, your hypothesis won't be confirmed until an autopsy is completed.

Accepting the second opinion was less of a problem than I thought it would be. *Okay, so, I have ALS. What now?* I already had gone through the deep depression by that point. So, how could I turn this situation around for my family and me? I refused to let the disease get the best of me. I remembered the fateful words of my favorite poet, Dylan Thomas: I wouldn't "go gently into that good night;" I would "rage, rage against the dying of the light,"[2] and be the most stubborn, salty bastard the disease had ever seen.

Don't get me wrong, more depression would rear its ugly head over the following year as I watched my body deteriorate before my eyes. Progression was quick and ruthless, showing no signs of stopping until it had taken all movement from my body. And the proverbial cherry on top was being ventilator dependent by the end of the year.

When I started researching what I could expect from the disease, I watched a lot of videos on the Internet about people who have ALS. These short documentaries scared the hell out of me.

The videos play hideous, sappy background music filled with sorrow and despair. They define what ALS is and tell us a little bit about the doomed victim: their age, first symptoms, date of diagnosis, etcetera. Next, the video digresses into a conversation about dealing with ALS. This part is accentuated by somber interviews with caregivers and family members, usually in tears, discussing how hard it is to see the patient wither away and die. Some videos go no further. But, if they really want to terrify us, they include more footage of the patient's ultimate demise. We see pictures of the emaciated patient staring into the camera through hollow, lifeless eyes.

I fell for it at first. Then, I was watching TV one night, and made the connection: those videos were no different than those rescued animal commercials. Conclusions I've come to from watching the "pound puppy" videos are: 1) this is not the image I want to project to the world – I will never make one of these videos; and 2) I would rather my wife leave me hanging naked like a human piñata in the Hoyer lift with my butt slathered in warm bacon grease over a pack of hungry raccoons than sit through another one of them.

I have ALS. Bear with me for just a moment; let's analyze the previous sentence. For the first couple of months after my diagnosis, I formed the nasty habit of saying "I have ALS." It didn't take long for me to start hating this sentence. To me, it meant I had surrendered to the disease, that I'd rendered myself dormant as ALS consumed all of me both mentally and physically.

Okay, good doctor, you're telling me I only have two to five years to live? *Screw you!* I'll show you a little something about the human spirit.

Oh, you say my quality of life will deteriorate if I get a trach? *Screw you twice!* Sit back and watch me live a fulfilling life. Maybe you'll learn something about what it means to really live.

That's right, I *live* with ALS. I choose to be positive. I choose not to give up. I look forward to waking up every day. I can't wait to be transferred to my wheelchair and sit in front of my computer to start my day. I choose to live every day to its fullest. I choose to live!

You can't see this passion because, on the outside, I'm motionless – a breathing statue. There are no signs of life except for the occasional yawn, a weak smile on my face, and the moment of recognition when my eyes fall upon yours.

ALS rarely affects the mind. I believe having this disease magnifies the strengths and weaknesses of your personality. Therefore, if you were a butthead in your pre-ALS life, there's a strong possibility you'll be more of a butthead after diagnosis. I'm the perfect example: it's fascinating the amount of trouble I can still get in-to.

It's chaos inside this head of mine, with untamed thoughts running wildly about. Like: who will I haunt first when I finally do go to the other side? Why does my dad insist on wearing that hideous comb over? What makes Lucky Charms™ so magically delicious? Does this lady who is trying to talk to me know she has a gigantic bat in the cave? Can somebody please get her a tissue?

My head is bursting with creative ideas; that's why I look forward to working at my computer. I can't wait to see what I'm going to come up with next: a new song, an idea for a video, or a short story concept begging to be explored.

I use eye-gaze technology made by a Swedish company called Tobii. Yes, the same country who brought you such entities as ABBA (Hey, don't laugh. You know you're rockin' "Dancing Queen" on your iPod), IKEA®, ultra-cool names like Bjorn and Sven, and one mighty tasty meatball. Tobii has restored morale and a welcome sense of individuality to quadriplegics around the world. This technology is invaluable to my wife, since it keeps me occupied and out of her hair. Without it, I would drive her absolutely crazy.

My Tobii allows me to do a bunch of cool stuff. For instance, it allows me to make music. The program I use is the perfect outlet for my musical creativity. It has virtual synthesizers, equalizers, awesome effects, and drum machines. This is right up my alley, since it allows me to tinker with different settings to come up with new, amazing sounds. If you knew how much I adore music, you would see how immersing myself in it is as close to heaven on earth as I can get.

I've made two videos so far: one for the ALS Association of Arkansas, and one for my song on iTunes. They're both on YouTube for your viewing pleasure.

My other creative outlet is writing short stories. What do I write about? Horror – I love horror. It's so intense that sometimes I prefer to read a scary story than watch my favorite sport (football). This intensity puzzles me because it blossomed after my diagnosis. I could pay a shrink to psycho-analyze my mind, only to tell me I have repressed memories of being chased around my house by the Kool-Aid man swinging an ax (or maybe that was the time I got a-hold of some bad smoke). Instead, I want to share my active imagination with you. Ghosts, goblins, witches, ghouls, and other things that go bump in the night are topics I'm not afraid to explore. If I'm not careful, I can stay up for hours thinking about the "what ifs," giving myself goosebumps in the process.

My point in telling you all of this is to show you that I do have a fulfilling life. I focus on what I can do, not what I can't do. ALS is not a death sentence. I still have goals to accomplish. After my diagnosis, my dreams didn't die they only got bigger.

Chapter 2 | Eating and Swallowing Problems in ALS

When the disease struck my mouth and throat, I lost the ability to eat and swallow safely. With stiff and weakened jaw muscles, eating became such a chore that it started to defeat its purpose – I burned more calories than I was taking in. Even though I was still eating solid food, I lost thirty pounds in four months. This is bad for someone with ALS, because I needed to take in a large amount of fat and protein to preserve as much muscle function throughout my body as long as possible.

For the first time in my life, doctors were ordering me to eat high-calorie foods – the good stuff. All my dreams had finally come true. Being a fat boy for my entire life, I didn't need to be told twice to eat anything I wanted. I tried to eat – I really did. But, when it takes 45 minutes to eat a small can of ravioli (a stark contrast to the boy who used to swallow cupcakes whole in junior high), there's a problem. I began to lose my appetite quickly because it became too hard to chew. How's that for karma.

I underestimated the nutritional needs I would have as a sedentary patient. The ALS clinic's nutritionist explained that I required at least 2,000 calories a day to sustain my body's normal functions. In my pre-ALS life I would've laughed at her and said, "2,000 calories? No problem. I can take care of that before lunch. Here, hold my beer – watch this." However, in my condition, it meant I would be eating all day just to meet my daily quota. I had no appetite what so ever, and the sight of food made me want to vomit. Talk about irony. Who says God doesn't have a mischievous sense of humor?

A choice had to be made: either maintain the current path I was on and likely die from aspiration pneumonia, choking, or malnutrition, or take the trail fewer people have traveled on, and live. The decision was a no-brainer for me; I opted for tube feedings.

Since I can't eat solid food anymore, I want to extend a special thanks to the countless number of chickens, cows, hogs, and turkeys who were sacrificed to feed me in my pre-ALS life. I assure you they have not died in vain. The size of my ass is proof their memory lives on.

Surprisingly, I don't miss food. Sure, I have my moments when a big, fat, juicy bacon cheeseburger appears on TV. I'm only human, and as it turns out, still a carnivore. But the moment passes quickly, because I remember how hard it was to chew one bite. Then I'll think about how long it would take to eat the burger; I conservatively estimate I could down the whole thing in just two hours, assuming I don't choke and die from eating it.

Holy cow! Two hours to eat a meal? Come to think of it, how much time did I waste in my lifetime eating? Going to a restaurant, waiting to be seated, deciding what to eat, hoping the server would stop messing around and take your order, and wondering why your food was taking so long to cook – I don't miss that. Now, my formula is hooked up to my feeding tube, turned on, and, voila, I'm feeding. I enjoy my extra time watching TV with my wife, reading, writing, and making fun of how other people eat.

I also was having difficulty swallowing, which introduced two problems to worry about: choking on my food and the possibility of aspiration pneumonia. Several muscles are at work during the act of swallowing; the largest one is the tongue. When the tongue atrophies, it can no longer dump food into the throat effectively. Furthermore, weakened muscles in the throat are not able to push the food farther down in to the esophagus. As food gets caught in the throat, blocking the windpipe, choking will occur.

ALS affects the epiglottis, the little flap on top of the esophagus that blocks food and liquid from entering the windpipe every time I swallow. As the epiglottis weakens, it fails to close properly causing leaks to form in its seal allowing these substances to enter the windpipe. The first time this happened, I was eating a powdered doughnut; everyone who has eaten these knows how easy it is to inhale the powdered sugar. Well, that's what happened to me. It threw me in to a terrible coughing fit.

A harsh reality everyone with ALS must face is that today is the strongest they will ever be. This fact is especially evident when you're watching your body's slow descent into complete paralysis. Adapting to this new norm means I must always think ahead of the disease. If I continued to eat and drink, the coughing spells, the possibility of choking, and developing aspiration pneumonia would only increase, while my ability to clear the airway would continue to diminish.

CHAPTER 3 | RESPIRATORY FAILURE IN ALS

In most cases of ALS, respiratory failure is the culprit responsible for patient deaths. *Wait a minute – earlier in this book didn't you say ALS attacks only the voluntary muscles?* This is correct.

We breathe all our lives without thinking about it. The act of breathing gets embedded into our subconscious, where it is interpreted as an automatic process. But we can stop breathing when we want to, then do an about-face and start breathing again when we choose. Therefore, the breathing process (and the muscles that control it) is voluntary.

The diaphragm is the muscle that enables us to expand and contract the lungs. As ALS weakens the diaphragm, the patient's ability to breathe is compromised. The first thing I noticed was that I couldn't inhale as deeply as I once could which also meant I wasn't able to hold those long notes when singing in the shower.

How was that possible? My diagnosis was only four months old, but the notorious death rattle of the disease had already come knocking at my door. Once my breathing was affected, I knew that was the beginning of the end. I was terrified.

A damaged diaphragm introduces a much deadlier issue, a silent killer that will sneak up on you if you're not careful: carbon dioxide poisoning. With a crippled diaphragm, the lungs cannot fully contract; and thus, they won't expel carbon dioxide adequately. The defective blood-gas exchange process allows carbon dioxide to build up in the bloodstream slowly and, if not properly treated, will result in carbon dioxide poisoning followed by respiratory failure.

The common symptoms of carbon dioxide buildup are dull headaches accompanied by drowsiness. These warning signs are subtle and can easily be mistaken for other ailments like allergies, a cold, or simple dehydration.

When you visit your local ALS clinic, the respiratory therapist (RT) will use a pulse oximeter to measure the oxygen saturation of the blood. A normal reading of 95-100% means your lungs are supplying the proper amount of oxygen to your body. However, the pulse-ox reading doesn't tell the whole story. For example, you may have a reading of 99%, but the carbon dioxide in your blood might be approaching lethal levels.

An *arterial blood gas test* (ABG) will sample the blood from the artery in your wrist to give you not only a more accurate pulse-ox measurement, but a clear indication of the carbon dioxide levels as well. If you are encountering regular dull headaches, especially if they are accompanied by fatigue, contact your RT or pulmonologist immediately. Urge them to perform an ABG test. If this test is beyond the capabilities of your ALS clinic, make an appointment with a pulmonologist.

Some confusion exists over what proper ventilation is for the ALS patient. In the case of patients with a non-functioning diaphragm putting them on oxygen would be a fatal error. For those who have sustained damage to the diaphragm, oxygen might appease them psychologically, but physically, the blood-gas exchange mechanism is still broken. Again, a normal pulse-ox reading will give a false sense of security. To properly ventilate a patient with ALS, the diaphragm must expand and contract fully, so proper blood-gas exchange can take place.

A strategy to preserve muscle function is currently the only course of action in ALS. One method in use today, which is designed to delay the onset of ventilator dependence, is the *diaphragm pacing system* (DPS). The patient must have working phrenic nerves (which control the diaphragm) to qualify for the device. The surgeon installs electrodes on the phrenic nerves that attach to an electronic pacing system outside the patient's body. When turned on, the pacing unit sends electrical impulses to the nerves, which stimulate them and tell the diaphragm when to function. The idea is to ration the usage of the diaphragm and prolong its life before the muscle succumbs to the effects of ALS. This device will not halt the progression of the disease.

The DPS method is highly controversial in its use. A recent study conducted in the United Kingdom in July of 2015 suggests the DPS is harmful to ALS patients. One reason for this may be the degenerative nature of the disease; if the phrenic nerve is intact when the DPS is installed, it's only a matter of time before ALS kills it, leaving a useless nerve. Another reason may be that stress from the surgery accelerates the effects of the disease. In fact, any trauma suffered by the afflicted body will expedite the process.[3]

In a 2016 press release announcing a new study involving the DPS, Synapse Biomedical Inc., the device's maker, stated "US experts argue that the UK results did not show pacing was harmful, rather that the use of DPS should be used in conjunction with NIV" (non-invasive ventilation).[4] Hey, if you don't like one group's findings particularly when it's bad news involving your product, question their credibility, then do your own trial in your lab with your equipment. It sounds like Synapse hates the rules of the game, so they're taking their ball and going home.

All sarcasm aside, I'm rooting for Synapse – I'm for anything that will improve the lives of ALS patients. If the data from the new trial supports safer standards for their product, so be it. Technology can always be improved upon.

At Christmas time in 2012 – the year of my diagnosis – when I was already wheelchair bound, I fell in my bathroom ending up in a jack-knife position with my right leg bent tightly between the tub and vanity. A couple of days later, blood clots from intensive bruising in my leg hit my lungs. The emergency room doctor told me they had never seen so many *pulmonary embolisms*

(PEs) scattered throughout both lungs. It turns out that blood clots are a danger the sedentary ALS patient must face. When a person has one PE, they struggle to breathe, and I had numerous; I should've died. My diaphragm was under tremendous strain while clearing the lungs of clots. As a result, my *forced vital capacity* (FVC) took a nose dive in the following months. Forced vital capacity is the measurement of the amount of air a person can forcibly exhale for as long as possible. Respiratory therapists use FVC statistics to keep track of the ALS patient's decline in breathing strength. Fortunately, one positive about ALS is that healthy lungs remain pliable and will respond to mechanical ventilation.

The bi-pap machine or *bi-level positive airway pressure* supplies positive pressure while the patient is inhaling and negative pressure when exhaling – it inflates the lungs, then sucks out the carbon dioxide. Additionally, the bi-pap has settings for both the inspiratory and expiratory parts of the breath. As the diaphragm wanes, these settings can be adjusted to make certain the patient's lungs inflate and deflate properly.

The bi-pap is designated for patients who use non-invasive ventilation – people who are ventilated through the mouth or nose. Various attachments can accomplish this: nose pillows, the "sip and puff" which enables the user to take a couple of breaths when needed, or a mask covering both the mouth and nose. I alternated between the nose pillows for daily use and the mask at night.

In my opinion, as soon as the RT determines the patient's breathing is being affected by ALS, they should start using the bi-pap. Most people need as much time as possible to familiarize themselves with the claustrophobic nature of wearing the mask and the new sensations that come with mechanical ventilation. When you've been breathing one way your entire life, then you introduce a new way of doing it to the brain, your mind will fight you every step of the way – at least mine did. The first few nights I slept with the mask, I endured a constant fear of suffocating in my sleep and panic induced by the false sense of air hunger my mind kept throwing at me. My wife put the pulse-ox on my finger, so I could see I was receiving air despite my body telling me otherwise. I had to repeat to myself, *Relax, I'm getting the air I need, everything is cool.* Of course, I had a choice: learn how to breathe with the bi-pap or face respiratory failure.

Non-invasive ventilation (NIV) has its limits, especially for me because I battled a nasty post-nasal drip brought on by chronic allergies. The resulting mucus settled in my lungs, making it tough for me to breathe. Since I had lost the ability to cough up secretions on my own, I had to rely on chest physical therapy, the cough assist machine, and suction to evacuate the mucus. The caveat with NIV, as I soon found out, was that clearing secretions through my mouth wasn't as effective as I thought it would be. My allergies were so awful that my family would routinely spend up to eighteen hours a day clearing my airway out until I could breathe comfortably again. Air hunger became my detestable companion, and blackouts were a perpetual threat.

That was no way to live. It was time to face the question which confronts every victim with ALS: do I want to extend my life by getting a tracheostomy? Or should I give up and take the easy way out? My answer was a resounding *Hell no!* Besides, I still had too much piss and vinegar running through my veins to throw in the towel and quit.

Chapter 4 | To Trach or not to Trach

Extending my life with a tracheostomy didn't present much of a dilemma for me. From day one I wanted to fight this disease with everything I could muster. That doesn't mean I don't have my share of doubts. To be honest, I'm still apprehensive after one of my acquaintances dies from this disease. I begin to ask myself, *Do these people know something I don't? Am I an idiot for choosing to live in a broken body? Am I a selfish ass for burdening my family with the stresses of ALS?*

But these episodes of self-doubt are always short-lived. They end when I look at my wife and see the love we have for one another, and when I wake up every morning knowing life is such a beautiful gift that I've been blessed with.

I informed my neurologist (a different one) of my decision to go through with the tracheostomy, but the one question I struggled with was this: How would I know the right time to get it? The neurologist was no help. Instead, they were more concerned with instilling the fear of God into my wife and me. The neurologist called us one afternoon; they said my quality of life would plummet, and they asked my wife was she prepared for the long days and nights caring for a husband chained to a ventilator through his trach?

Huh? I was physically exhausted from spending every waking moment of the last few weeks trying to clear out my lungs so I could take a couple of unimpeded breaths. I looked like a ghost from poor oxygenation. My quality of life had hit rock bottom, how could it get any worse? I was willing to take the chance.

The neurologist went on to tell us we could expect my life to last another six months to a year. What? I didn't know they could see into the future. They must have been consulting their Magic 8-ball® in the office. I have my own, but the most I can get out of it is, "Don't count on it" or "Reply hazy try again." Hmm. I bet they have the souped-up medical version, and with all those exact answers, that thing must be ginormous. It makes me wonder how I missed seeing it on all those visits to the doctor's office.

My wife and I weren't buying the negative rhetoric. And why the hell were we listening to a neurologist giving medical advice on the intricacies of the tracheostomy and mechanical ventilation anyway? That's like going into Victoria's Secret® for a jockstrap; it just doesn't work.

A couple of days later we notified the good doctor that we still wanted to go through with the tracheostomy. My neurologist wasn't happy about it but went ahead and referred us to a pulmonologist for a consultation. This is exactly what every neurologist should do when asked by an ALS patient about the trach or the vent. Do not pass go. Do not collect $200. Proceed directly to someone who specializes in the workings of the pulmonary system: a pulmonologist.

I went through the surgery under general anesthesia and with a 0% FVC. Immediately, my quality of life improved – what used to take eighteen hours now took only minutes. Cough assist and suction work so much better when you have a hole in your neck that enables you to go straight to the source of the problem. The color came back in my complexion, and I had the first good night of sleep since being diagnosed.

At the time of publishing, I have been living with the trach and vent for over three years. As far as being chained to a vent goes, this is not the case. I go to baseball games, concerts, football games, and Barnes and Noble®. I have traveled to such exotic locations as Perdido Key and the women's restroom at the Flora-Bama (the wheelchair took a wrong turn). Extending my life with the trach and mechanical ventilation was the best life choice I've ever made.

Okay, Kip, how do I know the trach is right for me? Allow me to answer with this observation: the desire to extend your life is directly proportional to your will to live. When is the right time to get the tracheostomy? I don't know the answer, but don't wait until you find yourself suffering from a serious bout of pneumonia. I waited too long to get mine. If my experience with life support has been good, then why don't more people with ALS choose to extend their life? That's a tough question to answer. I said earlier that ALS is one of the few diseases in which every patient treads a unique pathway as they progress through the disease. I'm talking about people in various stages of their lives – some old, some young, and some middle-aged – all with distinctive opinions and contrasting viewpoints.

There may be a person in their seventies who has lived a full life and is happy to let the disease run its course. At the opposite end of the spectrum sits a teenager, bright and curious, who is fascinated with discovering life's mysteries, their will to live unaffected by the disease. Somewhere in the middle is the victim diagnosed in their thirties, robbed of the active, thriving lifestyle they've led who now lies depressed in their hospital bed wanting badly for the nightmare to end. Next to them is the patient who isn't ready for the ride to end. They have adjusted well to the role fate has revealed, and they find beauty and tranquility in life's little subtleties every day.

The high costs associated with ALS is a factor a patient must think of when considering life support. In 2012, my power wheelchair cost approximately $28,000; my insurance at the time paid 80% which left me with a $5,600 co-pay. The price of my speech-generating device, which I can't do without, was $20,000 in 2013; Medicare chipped in 80% leaving a $4,000 co-pay (now that's a lot of bake sales). Furthermore, a $50,000 hospital bill with Medicare as your only insurance will yield a $10,000 out-of-pocket expense.

A patient with a trach and on ventilation must be within eyesight of a caregiver 24/7, 365 days a year. Hiring a private caregiver is an expensive endeavor; if you're going through a home health-care agency or hiring an RN, the costs will skyrocket. The spouse of the patient may quit their job to stay at home to care for the loved one, leaving them with no other source of income except the patient's disability check – if they even have disability insurance, that is. I certainly understand why patients facing these circumstances choose to opt out of life support.

Other patients lack the solid support system necessary for those who wish to extend their life. They may not have any relatives to call on to give them the requisite care and tender love needed to sustain their lives. Then, there are the patients who refuse to burden their respective families with the emotions and stresses that accompany ALS. Still, some patients are simply afraid of the tracheostomy and mechanical ventilation.

I would like to see more patients choose the trach; if we hung around longer then maybe we could draw greater attention to ALS. Sadly, some victims of this disease are in situations that make the idea of life support an impossibility. We who've chosen to extend our lives must be careful not to pass judgment on those patients who haven't. Regardless of their reasons, we shall hold their memory in our hearts with the utmost respect and will honor their brave struggle in our fight to end this deadly disease.

CHAPTER 5 | AFTER THE TRACHEOSTOMY

Patients living with the trach and mechanical ventilation must become aggressive and advocate for themselves if they want to survive. Hospitals and doctors will not call to check on the status of the patient, because, quite frankly, nobody outside of the patient's support system gives a damn if the patient lives. It's up to the patient to take the preventative measures that will decrease the likelihood of serious complications from forming due to poor maintenance.

Choosing a dependable, *durable medical equipment* (DME) provider for the patient's ventilation needs will lay a strong foundation for preventative care. Make sure the DME provider is available 24/7, 365 days a year to answer any questions the patient may have and, most importantly, respond to equipment emergencies. They should have a courteous and professional staff of RTs who visit monthly to check on you. If the RTs can't answer your questions, are unable to build a safe ventilation circuit, or are incapable of troubleshooting ventilation problems you may be having, it's time to find another provider, because your life is in danger. No, I'm not being overdramatic. Look, we live in a world where we depend on fallible machines to breathe for us, and the last thing we need is incompetence from DME providers.

I strongly advise against entering a hospice program. Its purpose is to provide palliative care for those patients who have reached the end of their lives. Hospice programs don't get paid if their patients improve; in short, they make money off people dying. As morbid as this sounds, death is a fact of life and the foundation on which the business is based.

The hospice programs I have dealt with paid for all my care, food (because I'm tube fed), and the medications needed to sustain life. To clarify, they billed Medicare for their services but wrote off the co-pay. A nursing assistant came in three times a week to bathe me; a nurse visited once a week to check my vital signs. Every three months, a doctor assessed my condition to see if I had regressed enough to remain on hospice. The help hospice provides, especially for an overwhelmed spouse, makes it awfully tempting for an ALS family to say yes.

Emergency room visits, emergency transport to the hospital, appointments with medical specialists, surgical procedures, and anything hospice deems as non-palliative care are not paid for. There's also a good chance you'll be kicked out if you indulge in any of these treatments – I'm proud to say I've been kicked out of two programs.

The first expulsion came after I'd decided to have the tracheostomy surgery. After the procedure, my quality of life improved dramatically, and I'm afraid complacency won out. Before we knew it, a year had passed us by. Our extensive research suggested the trach tube should be changed frequently. We began to make inquiries with the new hospice staff about the possibility of a trach change; as we suspected, their answer was an absolute "no." Then the question became: could we at least make an appointment with an ENT (ears, nose, throat) doctor for an evaluation of my trach site? We didn't get an answer right away. The request went up their chain of command where it bounced around between executive officers for a couple of weeks. Finally, an okay was given for a consultation with a pulmonologist; they were even going to make the appointment for us. That wasn't what we wanted, but it was at least an appointment with a doctor.

After a few months, hospice's attempts at scheduling an appointment were unsuccessful. The same trach had now been in my throat for a year and a half, and to make matters worse, the cuff was starting to fail (i.e., the cuff was becoming difficult to keep inflated, and it was filling up with moisture). The situation was critical; we had moved past the consultation straight to a trach change – we didn't have time to wait on hospice.

Decision time. Our options: we could go it alone and start advocating for ourselves, which also meant hospice benefits would stop, or we could stay under hospice, endure their lack of initiative while my condition deteriorated, and continue to have our financial burdens eased. Life or possibly death – that's what it really boiled down to. Of course, we chose life. Sure, we would face co-pays and bills, but how can you put a price on this beautiful gift called life?

Hospice programs offer valuable assistance to ALS families; for trached patients, though, it comes with a heavy price. I assume if you're thinking about the tracheostomy or have already received it, you have a lust for life. For the ALS patient this is synonymous with aggressive trach care. Use caution when entering hospice; make sure you understand the limits of the program, because professional intervention for your trach is inevitable.

—∽—

Trached patients are more susceptible to infections forming in the respiratory tract. Think about it: our breath enters a hole in the throat that leads directly to the lungs bypassing the body's natural bacteria filters – the mouth and nose. This is a problem for me because I've lost my sense of smell. I must rely on my four mothers (my wife, sister, caregiver, and RT) to tell me when an infection is imminent. They certainly don't sit around sniffing my trach like a fine wine connoisseur sticking their nose in a wineglass – that's just gross. But they do know when it's time to see a specialist.

Regular checkups – every six months – with an ENT doctor and a pulmonologist are also a substantial part of preventative care. The ENT is concerned with keeping the trach site free from infection. The pulmonologist specializes in ventilation and treating ailments in our lungs as they occur. Establishing a rapport with these professionals is a key element to surviving with the trach.

There's not much to a pulmonologist's office visit. Today's ventilators allow the patient to download their respiratory statistics and bring them along to give the pulmonologist an accurate picture of how the patient has been breathing in the past months. At the pulmonologist's, they ask how I'm breathing and if I'm experiencing unusual fatigue or headaches, check my vent statistics for any abnormalities, and swab the inside of my trach tube for a trach culture, this should be done at every checkup to see if the trach is clear of harmful bacteria. A chest x-ray and an ABG test are done annually.

Over time, the trach tube accumulates bacteria. Delaying a trach change allows the nastiness to increase, along with your chance of getting a serious infection. Another thing to consider is that the longer the trach stays in your throat, the more the surrounding trachea tissue will adhere to the trach. I went a year and a half without having my trach changed. I remember the first time the ENT changed the trach. After the change, heavy suction had to be performed to keep me from drowning in my blood. Then the doctor showed me the tube that had come out of me; it had green, fuzzy stuff hanging off it. I would've hated to examine the substance under a microscope; I'm afraid a new strain of bacteria might have looked at me and winked. The thought of those harmful microorganisms hanging around in my throat made me cringe. This was precisely the reason why I chose to have my trach tube changed out more frequently.

Trach tubes are divided in to two types: cuffed and uncuffed. The difference is that a cuffed trach, the kind I have, has a small balloon around its mid-section. When inflated, the balloon forms a seal that blocks air from escaping through the nose and mouth. You must be careful not to overinflate the cuff or abscesses in the trachea walls may form. If these sores aren't treated, the resulting tracheal erosion will eat through the windpipe causing air to seep out. Furthermore, one of these abscesses may even breach the tissue separating the trachea and esophagus, possibly allowing stomach acid to leak into the lungs. This was exactly what the ENT found while changing my trach tube. The abscess wasn't a deep wound, but it was severe enough to prompt further examination under general anesthesia. I emerged with a trach tube of a different length to prevent further eroding and to give the sore a better chance to heal.

An unfortunate side effect of a tracheostomy is the presence of granulomas. According to Google®, a granuloma is a mass of tissue the body grows in response to infection or a foreign substance being introduced into it. These growths don't form immediately after the surgery but may fester around the stoma and inside the trachea in the time following the operation. These can grow to a size that will affect the airflow in the trach tube, and, in some cases, the blockage may get so extreme that urgent emergency care is needed. If you have a granuloma, let your ENT know; let their expertise work for you. They will evaluate the growth and determine if surgery is required to remove it or if it can be treated with medication.

Chapter 6 | Passive Respiratory Therapy

Landing in a doctor's office or hospital with a medical problem that could've been prevented is not high on my bucket list. Good respiratory therapy habits can help me stave off ailments that could easily escalate into a life-threatening condition. The respiratory therapy I do is no guarantee against a bacterial infection or virus biting me in the ass someday, but I'm a big believer in making your luck and I'm convinced my therapy will soften the blow of the illness.

My passive respiratory therapy begins with protecting the lungs from disease and viruses through immunization. I always get an annual flu shot. Because the influenza virus mutates, the vaccine is not 100% effective. However, doctors say that if I do contract it, having the shot will decrease the severity of the infection. I received a bacterial pneumonia vaccine when I was diagnosed five years ago (I recently obtained the booster shot). This immunization shields me from the most common bacterium. I'm all for doing whatever it takes to increase my chance of survival.

My wife, Robin, performs trach care every day: she inspects the trach site and cleans around the stoma. Her examination includes monitoring the small granuloma growing out of my trachea; she is concerned with any significant change in size. Fluid, whether it's blood or mucus, always accumulates around my stoma and must be cleaned off. If it isn't, it will become entangled with my facial hair forming a stinky mass of hair and dried blood or mucus that's a breeding ground for unwanted bacteria. To prevent this, my wife shaves around the stoma once a week cleaning the dried gunk as needed.

Cuffed trach tubes come with an inner cannula. This is a small tube that fits inside the larger, outer trach tube. The sole purpose of the inner cannula is to serve as an emergency release when a plug occurs. In theory, removing the cannula will unclog the patient's airway. My wife and I have never put this to the test; we've always used the cough assist to get rid of plugs. Since the inner cannula rests inside the trachea, it also needs to be exchanged with a clean one on a regular basis. We change out my inner cannula at least twice a week; it's swapped out every day when I'm sick.

For those of us who use mechanical ventilation, hygiene doesn't stop at the trach site. The circuit tubes through which we breathe must be disinfected every week. Moisture from our breath and the in-circuit humidifier produces a warm, wet environment that bacteria love to flourish in. Robin alternates between two sets of circuit tubes each week: the set that is out of operation is soaked in Control III® disinfectant solution, so it's clean and ready to go for the next week. All circuit tubes should be replaced with new ones every three months.

As I stated earlier, airflow with a cuffed trach bypasses the mouth and nose. Not only do these serve as our body's natural filters for the air we breathe, but they also act as a humidifier warming and moistening the air for intake by the lungs. The cold, dry air blowing out of the ventilator will dry out the lungs raising the probability of plugs forming – think of them as boogers in your lungs, but larger and extremely dangerous.

To counter the development of plugs, artificial humidity becomes a necessity for mechanically ventilated patients. There are three methods of delivering artificial humidity to the trachea, with the first being the use of a room humidifier. Although the device will help raise the ambient humidity, which will indirectly improve conditions in your airway, it should not be viewed as the solution to the humidity problem. Instead, the room humidifier should supplement one of the following methods.

The next delivery method is a wire-heated, in-circuit humidifier. Ventilator air passes through the heated, moist environment of the humidifier and on to your lungs. I prefer this device because I can control the amount of heat it produces according to my needs. For example, if condensation develops in my vent tube – an indication that the humidifier is generating too much heat – I will cut back on the power. If my secretions are too thick or I feel like I'm too dry, I'll kick the humidity up a notch. Do not use ordinary tap water with this type of humidifier, only sterile water should be poured into its reservoir. Again, like everything else with the trach-ventilator circuit, it's important to disinfect the reservoir every week.

Use extreme caution when this in-circuit humidifier is in operation, because condensation will form in the vent tubes eventually. When an excessive amount of water collects in the vent tubes, the patient will sound like they're taking hits off a bong pipe or blowing bubbles in a glass of milk. When this happens, always disconnect the vent tube and empty accumulated water into a container – do not reuse this wastewater. Never, under any circumstances, let the water drain back into the patient's airway.

As we all know when water or any liquid is introduced into the lungs, it doesn't work out well for the patient. Pay attention!

The third and final method of adding artificial humidity into the circuit is the Heat Moisture Exchanger (HME). Also known as the artificial nose, this little gadget attaches to your vent tubes to become an in-circuit humidifier. The HME turns the heat from your breath into humidity. Its small size makes the apparatus portable and easy to travel with; I use it when I'm traveling long distances. The disadvantage of using the HME is that the power can't be adjusted according to your needs. They must be discarded every two to three days (during illness, it's recommended to change them out every day).

Warning: never use the wire-heated humidifier and the HME at the same time. This will create too much humidity. The surplus moisture will work its way into the sensitive electronics of the ventilator causing it to fail.

Chapter 7 | Active Respiratory Therapy

The sedentary nature of ALS puts the patient, especially one who's in the late stages of the disease, at a higher risk for developing pneumonia. Because of this lack of movement, fluid pooling in the lungs becomes another potentially life-threatening obstacle the patient faces daily. *Chest physical therapy* (CPT) can help with this problem. It consists of a series of exercises including various percussive techniques (clapping or tapping hands on the body) designed to break up mucus and induce the drainage of fluid out of the lungs.

One would think a guy who can't talk on his own would find it easy to stay out of trouble. I wish this were the case, but I've developed a knack for drawing my wife's wrath. How can a fully paralyzed, lovable man wreak more havoc than he did before he contracted ALS? I know, right? The point is, since I'm constantly on my wife's bad side, do I want to give her the opportunity to exorcise her Kip-frustrations in the form of percussive CPT? I don't think so. Some things are better left to the control of machines.

My CPT device employs *high frequency chest wall oscillation* (HFCWO) to accomplish much of what manual CPT does. The enacting of the machine's function takes place in an inflatable vest that I wear on my chest. It hooks to an air compressor via two hoses; controlled air bursts from the compressor, through the hose, and into the vest at a high frequency resulting in a rapid agitation of the chest wall. My routine consists of two ten-minute cycles: one at twelve hertz (Hz) and one at seventeen Hz, two times a day. Of course, if I'm battling a chest ailment, the sessions of CPT will increase.

It's important to expel the loosened mucus following a round of CPT with a cough assist machine. If you're able to cough effectively on your own, great, but if the disease has begun to affect your breathing, I suggest you start using the cough assist machine to help you eliminate secretions completely.

In my opinion, the cough assist is the one crucial machine that every ALS patient must have. It's saved my life more than a few times by dislodging plugs and giving me emergency ventilation when something had gone wrong with my ventilator. Also, regular usage of this machine has helped me ward off serious chest infections.

I was caught off guard when my feeding tube was placed, and I discovered my stomach had risen in my abdomen to the space previously occupied by the lower lobes of my lungs – they had decreased in size significantly. ALS had actually squeezed the breath out of me. I'm not saying this will happen to everyone with the disease (as we all know, ALS affects each person in different ways), but this does lead to another benefit of cough assist therapy: it hyperinflates your lungs which allows them to expand and contract completely.

Mechanical ventilation breathes for a patient within preset volume limits. Compared to normal breathing, mechanical ventilation is shallow in nature. Long periods of this soft breathing, without permitting the lungs to expand and contract fully, can cause the partial or total collapse of a lung – a condition known as *atelectasis*.

The cough assist machine inflates your lungs using a large burst of air on the inspiratory phase of the breath and pulls out debris on the expiratory phase. You are connected to the machine through a hose and a mask that fits over your mouth and nose (pre-trach). If you've had a tracheostomy, your DME provider will furnish a trach tube adapter connecting the trach to the hose. It takes a few sessions to get acclimated to the power of the device. The first few times I used it, I thought my eyes were going to explode out of their sockets like those unfortunate characters in cartoons. Be careful, because if your settings are too high, serious lung damage can occur. So, start with the settings at zero and work your way up to the levels you can tolerate.

I use the cough assist in times of stress when my respiration is too intense for my ventilator to keep up with. This frequently happens in football season; it's my favorite time of year. I love it all: high school, college, and pro – Canadian and American. My favorite teams won't play as I think they ought to, or a game comes down to the last play. My vent starts alarming, out comes the cough assist, and my wife threatens to turn off the game if I can't get it together. It's like clockwork; this happens every single time. I told you I stay in trouble. Seriously, though, just remember that if you feel anxious about your breathing, there's nothing wrong with taking a few deep breaths using the cough assist.

Having the power of the cough assist machine at your fingertips places a burden of great responsibility on your caregiver. You'll be astonished at how a simple, gooey ball of lung snot turns in to a weapon with deadly accuracy when a little charge of compressed air gets behind it. Beware: if your plugs are hard enough and your caregiver loses control of the hose, they might end up taking out a window or two.

There is always some residual mucus left over after my cough assist sessions. My caregiver uses the in-line suction to dispose of the lingering debris. The trachea and bronchial tubes are extremely delicate; you can easily nick a blood vessel with the suction tube causing the airway to bleed. This has happened to me before; the episode was so severe that it resulted in an emergency room visit. Because suctioning is so invasive, I prefer cough assist therapy to suction for clearing the majority of my secretions from the trachea.

Chapter 8 | Road Trips and Redundancy

Gone are the days when a patient was stuck inside the house tied to a ventilator. Today, thanks to technology, the trached and vented ALS patient can be as mobile as they desire. It's not uncommon to see them out on the town or on vacation, enjoying life, negating the myth that mechanical ventilation and the tracheostomy will cause your quality of life to suffer dramatically.

Every time I venture out in public, it feels like I need a tractor-trailer rig to follow me around carrying all the auxiliary equipment I require in case of an emergency. The equipment I take with me includes: my Tobii SGD, the ventilator, the cough assist, a portable suction machine, one Ambu bag, and various bandages and supplies. I'm easy to spot – look for a massive, white, bald head with a black headband and thick glasses. Robin will be driving the wheelchair with my caregiver in hot pursuit dragging a cart full of necessities. I think my entourage is overkill sometimes, but we can't afford to let our guard down. We always prepare for the worst and hope for the best.

We've traveled away from home a few times. Our largest excursion was to the beach in Florida – a ten-hour drive. My ventilator can carry two three-hour batteries for a total of six hours of breathing time. It seemed we had a slight discrepancy in the numbers. Since I wasn't interested in holding my breath for four hours, I thought it best to do a little research on powering the essential medical devices in our van.

We bought a car adapter for the ventilator, so it could run on the van's juice. Both the cough assist and the suction machine had limits on their batteries, but the suction machine had a deeper issue. When operating on battery power, it couldn't handle the load placed on it by the deep suctioning of my lungs.

While researching a solution, I came across someone who ran a ventilator off a car battery and a power inverter. I don't think so. There's no way I was having an exposed car battery with wires running everywhere in the back of the van. I graduated with a bachelor's in electronics engineering; I've worked with electricity over the years. When my old lab partner chased me down and zapped me with a wire that had 120 volts coming out of it ("C'mon, Kip. Be a man, it'll only sting for a bit."), I felt the raw bite of untamed electricity and have respected it ever since. For the record, I crossed him off my Christmas card list years ago.

I settled on an *uninterrupted power supply* (UPS) for my power solution. I remembered these nifty accessories from my not-so-proud days in the information technology field. The UPS prevents your computer from rebooting when the lights flicker, and more importantly, during long power outages it gives you the opportunity to shut it down properly, decreasing the chance of a sudden power loss corrupting your system. Batteries within these apparatuses make it possible for the UPS to do its job.

I liked the UPS because it was less cumbersome than a car battery, plus it had power receptacles so my caregiver could plug in the desired machine cleanly without any loose wires. A ninety-minute charge is what I get from my UPS, which, compared to a car battery, is not much. But with my ventilator running off the van battery, the only reason I would need the UPS was to run the cough assist and suctioning machine for five minutes a session. At that rate, the low battery capacity was much more attractive.

Get ready to shell out some green for a UPS. You can't get away with buying the cheapest model either. A UPS can output one of two types of power: simulated or pure sine wave. Here's where I'm just itching to geek out on you and explain the science behind both types of outputs, but I'll graciously refrain from indulging in my nerdiness. Think of simulated sine wave output as dirty power; devices that run off this output tend to run hot while fighting the noise produced by the power supply itself, which can interfere with the proper function of the machine. Pure sine wave output, then, is clean power, the type of UPS I use to run my sensitive medical equipment. These power supplies are more expensive than their less efficient counterparts, but it's worth the extra expense knowing my devices are running on cleaner power.

The same principle may be applied when shopping for back-up generators. I don't like to think about catastrophes, but it's a reality we all must face. Routine maintenance and testing are vital to a generator to make sure it can be started when needed. You should start your generator every week; however, if you choose not to do this, don't let fuel sit in the tank for long periods of time, because gasoline will become ineffective if it's not used.

Ventilator failure is always a possibility; it's a chilling scenario straight out of my nightmares. In my back-up plan, I will use the cough assist for emergency ventilation and, if this machine fails, I will fall back on the Ambu bag. Regardless of whether we think we have control of the situation, EMS will be called to lend assistance. You can never have too many hands when bagging a patient. Besides, it keeps my options open: if the DME provider will be there quickly with a replacement ventilator, everything's groovy, but if my vitals start to crash, I can be rushed to the emergency room.

Chapter 9 | Close Encounters of the Kip Kind

Don't be afraid to come up and say hello when you see me out in public. By the way, I'm totally aware of my appearance – I look like the product of an experiment gone awry when little Jimmy played with his first chemistry set ("Hey, mom! Look what I did."). Aside from my entourage, the machines, the tubes sticking out of me, the wheelchair, and my face, which is frozen in an idiotic stare complete, with a tiny stream of drool trickling down my chin (oddly enough, this is how I looked before the disease),

I'm a regular person just like you. I won't bite – I swear. Just remember to keep your fingers and hands away from my mouth at all times and there shouldn't be any problems.

I can't decide whether it's my feeble-minded gaze or my wheelchair or both that bring out the stupidity in people. They assume because you're severely disabled you're deaf. They bend over until their face is in front of yours, then proceed to yell out every word slowly while they over-enunciate every syllable showering you with spit on every consonant. Oh, my God! Will someone get this moron out of my face? I can hear perfectly, and if anybody is the fool in this conversation, believe me, it's this igmo trying so desperately to hold a conversation with me. No, I'm not paying attention to you, I'm thinking of exciting ways to run you over in my wheelchair.

When one or more of your senses become incapacitated (my smell and taste), I believe your body compensates by making the remaining senses stronger – I hear and see a hell of a lot more than you think I do. I hear the "retard" comments; I see the adults who snicker and stare. My parents raised me better. If they'd seen me act the same way, the first thing mom would've done was to slap me silly, and then dad would've knocked me into next week.

I made a promise to myself when I was diagnosed that I would never be ashamed to go out in public. So, what about the gawking lowlifes who laugh at the unfortunate plight of their fellow human beings? I say, piss on 'em! For every one of those goobers, there are hundreds of people who see God's light shining through me. If the sight of me causes someone to hug their spouse a little tighter or kiss the kids more often thanking God for their healthy family, I don't have a problem with that.

EMTs, firefighters, paramedics, and police officers: listen up. When you respond to a trached and vented ALS patient's residence, chances are it's because the patient is in respiratory distress of some kind. Possibly the best strategy for stepping into this foreign environment is to yield to the caregiver's authority – they are in charge. The caregiver is more familiar with the machines the patient uses, particularly when interpreting their alarms. It's this knowledge that will help you determine if the root cause of the problem is an equipment malfunction or trouble with the patient's airway. When transport is required, I suggest allowing the caregiver to ride in the back of the ambulance with their patient, because the caregiver will be able to communicate more effectively with them, especially under nonverbal circumstances. A situation might occur in which the patient's ventilator is working, yet they keep blinking, clicking their teeth, or grunting furiously at you. Without the caregiver present, you wouldn't know whether the problem is as simple as a comfort issue, or something more serious like a blocked airway (just because the vent looks like it's working, that doesn't necessarily mean the patient is receiving good airflow).

Nurses, I love you. I have the ultimate respect for everyone who chooses the profession. A sick human being is not a pretty sight, and dealing with one takes a dedicated, caring soul. ALS attacks every single voluntary muscle in your body; it has disfigured my face depriving me of the ability to make facial expressions (I can still manage a weak smile). If I'm angry, I have a blank face. If I'm shocked, it's the same blank stare. If I think you're sexy, there's no change. Therefore, it's hard to tell when you're hurting me because, of course, my appearance will not waver. I can't yell out in pain, and my muscles don't work, so there's no reflex in response to stimuli. A good rule to follow with me or any fully paralyzed, nonverbal ALS patient is that if the action would hurt you, I guarantee we're in pain.

Unfortunately, in hospitals, progress is held up waiting on doctor's orders to come through, and since I have a feeding tube, this waiting complicates things. Where normal patients may have water any time they desire, I must wait for orders. This sucks, because the longer I go without water, the more things dry out causing further problems. If you happen to see me taking in water before the physician's orders arrive, have a heart and look the other way.

All medical personnel, be advised: Robin and I do stuff that may seem out of the ordinary, but it gets the job done – we know what works. We've been at this a lot longer than you've been a part of our lives. Please remember this when caring for all ALS patients.

Picture this: you're in the middle of patient rounds. You step out into the hallway. From the end of the corridor, a hideous din of noise bounces off the walls and into your ears. Your watch reads 8:18 a.m. *What on God's green earth could that be?* you wonder, as you search for the source of this audible anomaly. Your gait quickens as the sound becomes almost unbearable. There's only one room left; could this be the origin of the commotion? You're in front of the door, now. The noise is starting to take on form. Heavy guitars are strumming along to the thick beat of drums. A high, piercing voice screeches its way through the lyrics. Then you pick up on an even louder voice saying, "Kip, turn that crap down!"

You open the door to see my wife yank my computer away from me and start pushing buttons trying desperately to shut my music off. I've got a weak smile on my face. Though you're not sure, you swear I'm laughing my ass off at her. Robin finally succeeds in turning off my music, but not before she hurls a derogatory comment my way. Welcome to my room.

Everything I do centers around my SGD. It speaks for me. I can surf the net, keep up with social media, and play my music – loud. My SGD has an obnoxious alarm on it; I've only had to use this once when a nurse took it upon herself to catheterize me unnecessarily. I turned up the volume and let her have it. It got her attention, too. Don't put things inside my body, especially where it's exit-only, unless permission is specifically granted by me. This goes for all medical personnel. You've been warned.

I'm excited to show you my SGD. I'll even let you come look over my shoulder as I type. Speaking for myself, I don't mind if you finish my sentences before I do. The more you guess correctly the less I need to type. Please remember that other patients might not feel the way I do, so please respect their wishes.

Ah, the things you learn about your family in desperate times. For instance, I found out a few close relatives were mouth breathers (literally). I detest being breathed on; you have no idea how many times I've been coughed on, sneezed on, and spit on ("If I had a quarter for every time..."). Now, I know, nurses and respiratory therapists, it's impossible – due to the close proximity to the patient required by your occupations – to hold your breath or stifle a sneeze every time you interact with one of us, but you should be aware of your health at all times. Glove up, and if you've got a case of the sniffle-snorts, no matter how small, please wear a mask. Remember, a simple cold for you could very well be the death of us patients.

Finally, respiratory therapists, this one's for you. Previously I discussed the power of the cough assist machine. When administering cough assist therapy on me, please watch where you point that thing when you're emptying it. The last thing I want is to be hit in the face with my own snot rockets. I don't care if you let it rip hitting my relatives across the room (aim for the open mouths). Do everything in your power to keep my lung boogers from hitting me. Thank you, in advance, for your cooperation.

Afterword

I won't say that writing this book has been therapeutic for me, but it has allowed me to step out of the patient persona and assume, albeit quite briefly and lacking the extensive medical training, the perspective of the neurologist. Having said this, it's important to know that my interpretations and opinions of the encounters with neurologists depicted in this book are mine alone.

Final judgment should be reserved until every viewpoint has been thoroughly examined. I could not in good conscience close this book without considering the circumstances in which neurologists work every day. What if I had to inform a human being of their impending death from a disease that, despite years in medical school and residency and my vast experience in neurology, I'm helpless to stop? How would I respond if I witnessed patient after patient slowly withering away and dying for years knowing I could do nothing to halt the disease's progress? What would've become of me if I was living this scenario? I know exactly what would've happened: I would've become a calloused, pitiful excuse for a man with Mr. Jack Daniel as my only friend.

Enduring this kind of sadness demands a resilience seen in few individuals. This is a person who manifests enormous strength in order to absorb the emotional blows to their psyche, pushing through with a driving tenacity, determined to find the elusive cure for this horrible disease.

As for me, these qualities form the solid foundation of my faith that neurologists will find a cure for ALS in my lifetime. Until then, I'll be hanging out watching football, writing trash horror stories, enjoying life with family and friends, and waiting on my free pudding voucher to be delivered.

Works Cited

1. The ALS Association. (n.d.). What is ALS? Retrieved from http://www.alsa.org/about-als/what-is-als.html
2. Thomas, Dylan. (1938). Do not go gentle into that good night. Retrieved from https://www.poets.org/poetsorg/poem/do-not-go-gentle-good-night
3. Dance, Amber. (2015). Study Suggests Respiratory Pacemaker Reduces ALS Survival. Retrieved from http://www.alzforum.org/news/research-news/study-suggests-respiratory-pacemaker-reduces-als-survival#show-more

4. Synapse Biomedical Inc. (2016). New ALS Device Trial; the PARADIGM Study Will Continue Research of the NeuRx® Diaphragm Pacing System (DPS) in ALS Patients. Retrieved from https://www.prnewswire.com/news-releases/new-als-device-trial-the-paradigm-study-will-continue-research-of-the-neurx-diaphragm-pacing-system-dps-in-als-patients-300323247.html

FOLLOW MY BLOG AT:

WWW.KIPLINGAJACKSON.COM

Help ALS patients now!
Donate to your local
ALS Association chapter:

ALSA.ORG/COMMUNITY/CHAPTERS/

Made in the USA
Middletown, DE
07 April 2018